COMMUNITY HEALTH INSURANCE

AGENTS TRAINING

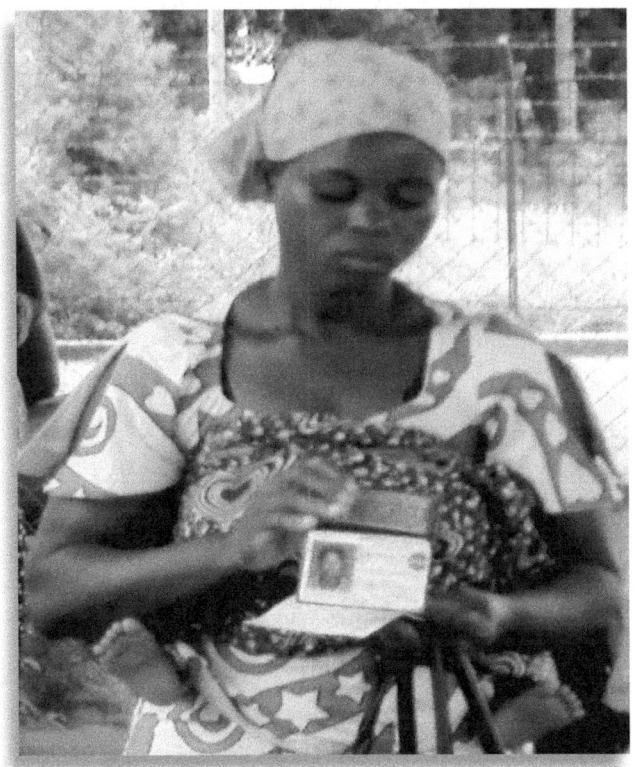

Key to Sustaining Pro-Poor
Access to Health Care in Ghana

1. Executive Summary

The creation of wealth and opportunities to reduce the worse forms of poverty, hunger and disease in developing countries especially led to the formulation of the Millennium Development Goals (MDGs) in 2000.

In Ghana, making health services accessible and affordable for all citizens engaged the attention of government and stakeholders following the operationalization of the MDGs. As a result of the intensive discussions ad consultations, the National Health Insurance Policy was formulated and rolled out in all districts in the country.

National Health Insurance is manned by District Mutual Health Insurance Schemes at the Metropolitan, Municipal and District Assembly levels. A Regional Coordinating Unit supervises all mutual health insurance schemes in each of region while the

National Health Insurance Authority (NHIA) oversees all health insurances activities in the country.

The facilitation of SNV-Netherlands Development Organization has brought a lot of the challenges faced by Mutual Health Insurance Schemes in the Upper West Region. Most of their challenges exist because of capacity gaps of Community Health Insurance Agents (CHIAs) in participatory community mobilization, indigent identification, facilitation, and resource mobilization. Other factors include the low staff strength of schemes and inadequate expertise in clients' handling.

SNV therefore contracted Center for Community Participation and Development, a local NGO with great expertise in community mobilization, as a Local Capacity Builder to train CHIAs in Wa Municipal and Sissala West District. In all, one hundred and seventy (170); 56 in Wa Municipal and 114 in Sissala West participants were trained on effective ways of mobilizing their communities and identifying indigents.

Participants described the training as being very effective and participatory. They were impressed with the training package and delivery. Therefore, participants acquired important skills especially, on who an indigent is and how to identify him/her. Resource mobilization using the Village Savings and Loans Associations concept was another key point that participants picked along.

LIST OF ACRONYMS

CCPAD	Centre for Community Participation and Development
CHIAs	Community Health Insurance Agents
FGDs	Focus Group Discussions
GPRS	Ghana Poverty Reduction Strategy
LCB	Local Capacity Builder
LI	Legislative Instrument
MDGs	Millennium Development Goals
MOH	Ministry of Health
NGO	Non-Governmental Organization
NHIA	National Health Insurance Authority
NHIS	National Health Insurance Scheme
NSD	Network for Sustainable Development
PRO	Public Relations Officer
SNV	Netherlands Development Organization
SWDMHIS	Sissala West District Mutual Health Insurance Scheme

VSLAs   Village Savings and Loans Associations

VSLS   Village Savings and Loans Scheme

WMHIS   Wa Municipal Health Insurance Scheme

Table of Content

<u>Tables</u>

2. Introduction

The development of poverty reduction schemes has engaged the attention of all states especially after the United Nations Millennium Summit (UNMS) in 2000, which produced the Millennium Development Goals (MDGs). The overall aim of the MDGs is to reduce the incidence of poverty by 2015

Following that, Ghana developed the Ghana Poverty Reduction Strategies (GPRS I and GPRS II) to localize the MDGs and to work in a more coordinated way towards their achievement. A number of schemes and programmes are borne out of the GPRS I & II and are contributing to the attainment of the MDGs. The National Health Insurance scheme (NHIS) is one of such schemes setup by Act 650 (2003) to address the problem of financial barriers to health care access within the context of the Ghana Poverty Reduction Strategy (GPRS)[1].

---

[1] MOH 2004, National Health Insurance Framework Policy for Ghana, Revised Version

The policy objective is to initiate a National Health Insurance Scheme (NHIS), which will ensure that, "within five years, every resident of Ghana will belong to a health insurance scheme that adequately covers him or her against the need to pay out-of-pocket at the point of service". The ultimate vision of the government for instituting the health insurance scheme in the country is to assure equitable and universal access for all residents of Ghana to an acceptable quality package of essential health care[2].

Per the National Health Insurance Act (Act 650) and Legislative Instrument (LI) 1809 (2004), the national health insurance authority, district mutual health insurance schemes and private health insurance schemes have been setup. The LI further mandates the establishment of the General Assembly made of community level stakeholders including the Community Health Insurance Agents. This is in appreciation of the enormous role community

---

[2] Balancing Access with Quality Healthcare: An Assessment of the NHIS in Ghana (2004-2008), SEND Ghana, May, 2010

stakeholders have in the porvision of quality health insurance.

Since 2003, health insurance in Ghana has gone through series of fine-tuning and capacity building of the sort at the national, regional, district and community level to increase enrolment and enhance service delivery. That notwithstanding, the scheme with facilitation from SNV – Netherlands Development Organization identified the need to train community health insurance agents on participatory community mobilization techniques for them to effectively work well in their communities.

Following that, CCPAD, a local NGO with expertise in community mobilization, was contracted by SNV – Netherlands Development Organization to design training materials and train community health insurance agents in Sissala West, Wa East Districts, and Wa Municipal, all in the Upper West Region. The assignment spanned from October 2009 to June 2010.

As part of many other things, this report intends to provide information on partners to facilitate the better understanding of an outside reader. It also seeks to clearly outline the outcomes and indicate the possible impact of the assignment.

3. Background of CHIA Training

The introduction of the National Health Insurance Scheme comes with the good intention of creating access to health care for the poor who could not easily do so under the cash and carry system. However, its implementation has revealed a lot of challenges that is rolling back the possible gains of the scheme. Though challenges such as inadequate human resource, inadequate equipment and weak management systems are national in nature and are common to all schemes, there are other challenges that are specific to individual schemes. Therefore, in addressing the challenges to better the service delivery situation, there is the need to have different intervention approaches to take care of:

1. National level challenges

2. Regional level challenges

3. Common challenges of District Mutual Health Insurance Scheme

4. District Mutual Health Insurance Schemes' specific challenges

With that understanding and working through its intervention approach of providing capacity building and facilitating processes for improvement, the health team of the Upper West portfolio of SNV-Netherlands Development Organization first conducted an exploration of all schemes in the Upper West Region to identify their capacity gaps and areas that they needed technical support. Significant among the many outlined challenges was the issue of mobilizing communities effectively for health insurance.

It was realized that community level structures, such as the community health insurance committees, were not working effectively to conduct the needed mobilization for health insurance. That has resulted in low coverage in most instances. Also, as a result of the capacity gap in the area of community and resource mobilization, health insurance agents were not able to present to community members alternative ways of paying premium that conveniently fitted into their context to make premium payment more effective.

All schemes therefore indicated the need to have their structures at the community level trained on participatory community mobilization to enable them enroll many more people. The second objective of undertaking participatory community mobilization training was also to equip community health insurance agents with skills and strategies to aggressively reach out to many more indigents. With such a move, schemes expect to improve the level of social mobilization which will positively show in an increased enrolment into the various schemes.

SNV therefore supported the schemes by engaging the services of organizations with in-depth experience in participatory community mobilization to deliver training for community health insurance agents while the schemes contributed the other component of the training cost. Centre for Community Participation and Development (CCPAD) and Network for Sustainable Development (NSD) were contracted first to develop training materials based on identified training topics in collaboration with the respective schemes and SNV, and also to deliver the training.

Centre for Community Participation and Development was assigned to deliver the training in Wa Municipal and the Sisaala West District. This report is based on the training conducted in the above districts.

4. How Assignment Fits Into Health Insurance

The participation of community members (beneficiaries) in health insurance is very relevant in ensuring ownership and sustainability. Right in the centre of focus of all mutual health insurance schemes is the beneficiary. The Public Relations unit headed by the Public Relations Officer (PRO) initiates and implements strategies that will promote more public participation in the activities of the scheme.

As part of ensuring more participation of community members in the processes, Community Health Insurance Agents (CHIAs) are identified and supported to engage community members in health insurance issues. Importantly, CHIAs are to design and present messages that will draw many more people to join health insurance in their respective communities.

Therefore, capacity building for CHIAs is a very important ingredient in the work of health insurance, especially in the area of participatory methodologies. The objective of the assignment clearly satisfies the need for efficiency in community mobilization. It seeks to sharpen the skills of CHIAs and staff of mutual health insurance schemes to effectively mobilize communities for health insurance.

5. Briefs on Partners

A. The Wa Municipal Mutual Health Insurance Scheme

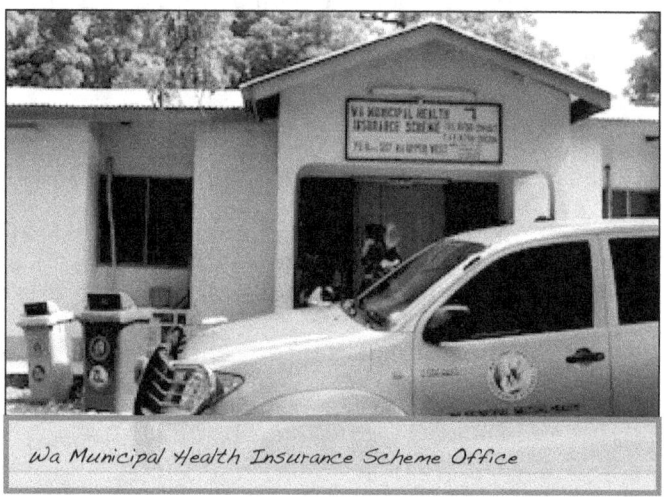

Wa Municipal Health Insurance Scheme Office

The Wa Municipal Health Insurance (WMHIS) was created by the health insurance act of 2003. It started operation in 2001 as one of the 45-piloted schemes in the country. Until 2006, when Wa East and Wa West schemes were carved out, a focal person was managing it. Currently, the scheme has a four-tier management structure comprising the General Assembly, The Board of Directors, the Management Team, and the CHIAs.

The scheme operates mainly in the Wa Municipality which hosts the regional capital, Wa. It serves about 72 communities with an estimated population of 113,954. 52.84% located in the Wa Township.

Apart from serving the Wa municipality, people from other districts such as Wa West, Wa East and Nadowli districts subscribed to the scheme because the regional hospital and prominent pharmaceutical outfits are located in the municipality. In recent times that has changed with the coming into being of the national health insurance card which allows people to access health service in any health facility in the country.

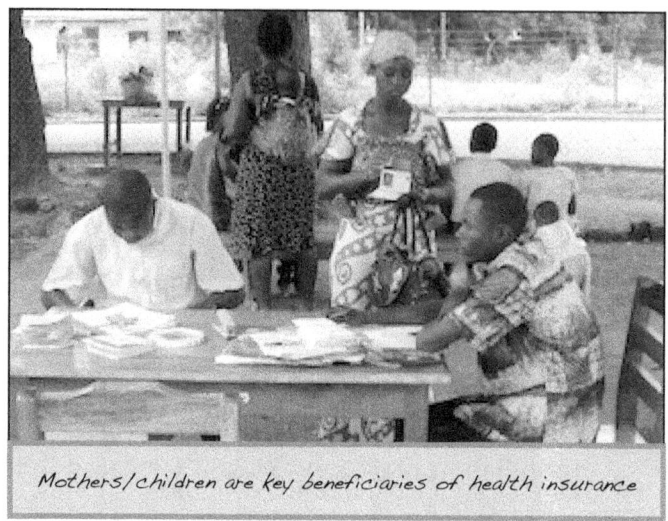

Mothers/children are key beneficiaries of health insurance

In terms of enrolment, the trend has been changing right from 2001. From 2001 to 2005 increase in enrolment was steady. However, as a result of progressive and radical public sensitization embarked upon by the scheme, the number of people enrolled increased from 26,534 (24.06% of population) in 2005 to 55,310 (50.13% of population) in 2006. In 2008, 87% of the population had been covered[3].

---

[3] 2008 Annual Report of Wa Municpal Health Insurance Scheme.

B. The Sissala West District Mutual Health Insurance Scheme

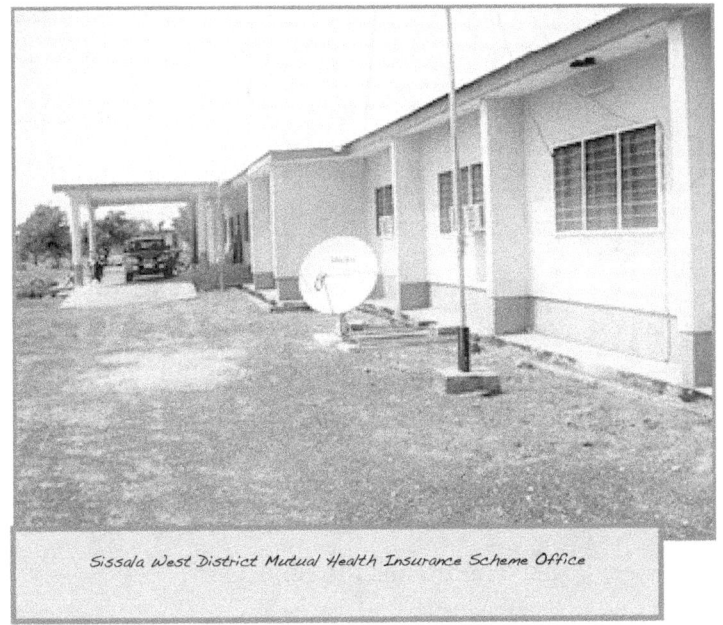

Sissala West District Mutual Health Insurance Scheme Office

The Sissala West District Mutual Health Insurance Scheme (SWDMHIS) was established in 2006 as part of the national policy framework, which provides for the establishment of Mutual Health Insurance Schemes in all Districts in the country. The mandate of the scheme rests on the National Health Insurance Act 650 of 2003 and LI 1809 of 2004.

The population of the district was 44,440 in 2000 according to the 2000 population and housing census, and has an estimated population growth rate of 1.7%. In 2005, the District Administration estimated the population of the district at 51,015 based on the growth rate. Using the growth rate and 2005 as the base year, the expected population of the district is 54,573 for 2010.

However, 23% of the population are active members of the scheme though the percentage could be higher when one looks at all enrolments.

The scheme has the objects of:

a. Increasing current level of active membership of 23% to 80% in 2014

b. Acquiring permanent office accommodation of the scheme by 2012

c. Enhancing collaboration with stakeholders by 2014

These objectives are contained in the schemes five-year strategic plan (2010-2015). SNV –

Netherlands Development Organisation through her health advisor Remy Nyewie, facilitated the development of the strategic plan.

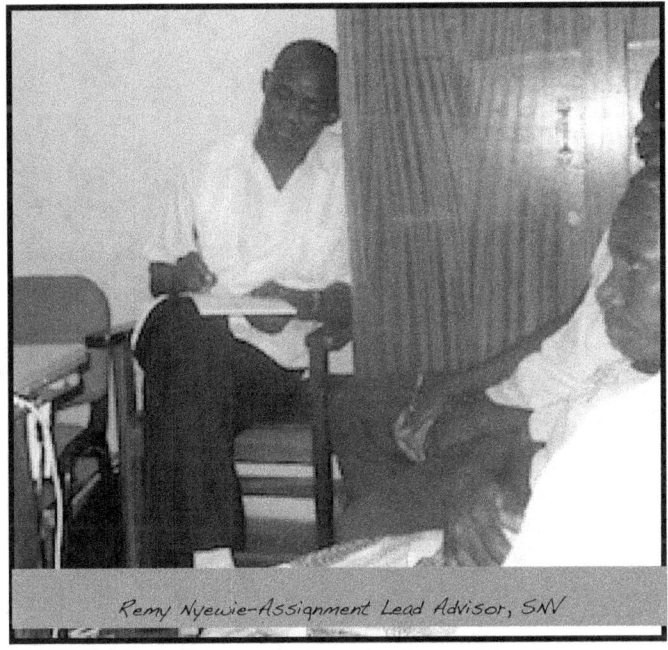

Remy Nyewie-Assignment Lead Advisor, SNV

With the achievement of the objectives, the scheme will be able to better serve many more people in the district. The objectives are contained in the schemes strategic plan 2010-2015

C. SNV-Netherlands Development Organization

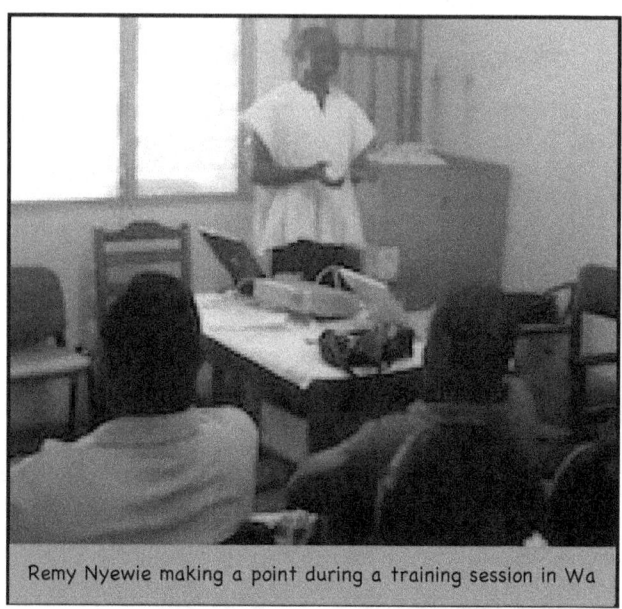

Remy Nyewie making a point during a training session in Wa

SNV – Netherlands Development Organisation is a Dutch Government funded non-profit, international development organisation, established in the Netherlands in 1965. SNV has been operating in developing countries for over 40 years and now operates in 35 countries in Africa, Latin America and the Balkans. Its focus areas are Education, Health, Renewable Energy, Water and

Sanitation, Agriculture, Forestry, Tourism and Inclusive Business.[4]

The Upper West Portfolio, opened in December 2008, operates in the region with focus on

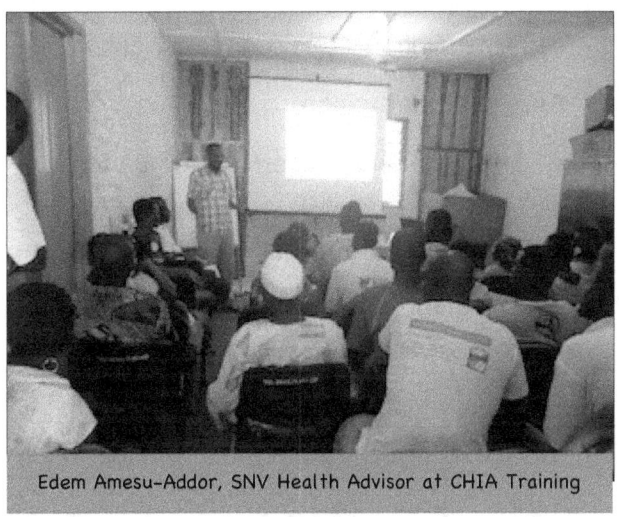

Edem Amesu-Addor, SNV Health Advisor at CHIA Training

Education, Health and Local Economic Development through Shea.

The Health component has focused on improving Health Insurance as the first activity in health. All the schemes in the region have been explored and a number of activities have been carried out.

---

[4] SNV website: www.snvworld.org

Significant among them is the support given to five (5) schemes to develop strategic plans. Through this, schemes have developed road maps that will improve health insurance in their respective district. Also, SNV has supported capacity building of Community Health Insurance Agents on participatory approaches in community mobilisation and indigent identification.

D. Centre for Community Participation and Development

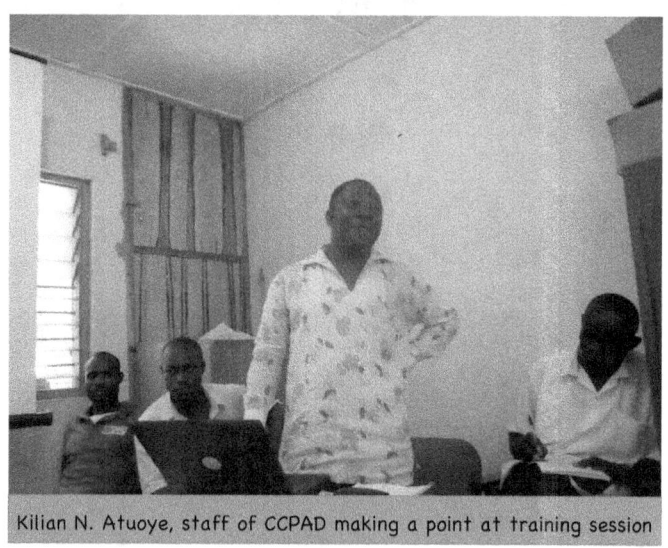

Kilian N. Atuoye, staff of CCPAD making a point at training session

Center for Community Participation and Development is a non-governmental organization formed in 2009 to respond to the immediate need for a competent local NGO to undertake participatory community mobilization.

CCPAD is focused on Education, Health, Agriculture and Livelihoods using community mobilization, advocacy, and capacity building/training. CCPAD aims at effectively implementing interventions that seek to reduce poverty, inequality, illiteracy and unemployment, and promote ownership among local communities with strong grounding on the philosophy that local communities understand their own problems better and have better solutions.

The organization has a well-developed structure that informs its smooth running. It has a Board of Directors, the Management Team and community level volunteers. All staffs have in-depth knowledge on focus areas and the strategies of the organization, though they come from different professional backgrounds. That makes the team multi-disciplinary and more effective in undertaking activities and programmes in the focus areas.

6. How the Assignment Was Carried Out

The assignment was conducted under two main headings. First was the development of training materials. In consultation with SNV and the schemes, training topics were identified. Following that, CCPAD and NSD worked together to develop the training materials and SNV validated them. In designing the training materials we took into consideration the training environment, the educational levels of participants and the profiles of the communities that participants were coming from in order to have a more participant-centered training material.

The second aspect of the assignment was the training it self. In both Wa Municipal and Sissala West, the training was conducted in batches because of the high number of CHIAs that the training targeted. Each batch was given a two-day training. In all, 12 days were used to effectively conduct the training.

The training was conducted using participatory methodologies such as group work, power point presentations, demonstration, brainstorming and open forum. Icebreakers were commonly used to energize participants throughout the training. Expansion of the entire training process is done below.

A. Pre-Assignment Activities

Before the signing of contract between CCPAD and SNV-Netherlands Development Organization, several important activities took place including:

1. Exploration meetings

2. Development and Discussion of Expression of Interest (EoI)

3. Development and Discussion of Technical Proposal and Budget

4. Contract Design and Signing

First of all, two exploration meetings were held between the health team of the Upper West Portfolio of SNV and CCPAD in 2009. The objectives of the meetings were to understand what each organization does and also identify possible areas of collaboration. Significant also, was to appraise the capacity of CCPAD in terms of staff strength, logistics and experience. It was quite easy because CCPAD had earlier presented her profile to SNV, which clearly indicated all the above areas.

Based on the success of the exploration discussions, another meeting was organized during which SNV indicated what was planned for health insurance and requested for an expression of interest in that regard which was appropriately submitted by CCPAD

Further discussions were done on the expression of interest after which a technical proposal was developed and submitted to SNV. Based on assessment of the proposal by SNV, a meeting was held to allow the two organizations to discuss the technical proposal and the budget.

Following the discussion on the technical proposal, the decision was taken to award a Local Capacity Builder (LCB) contract to CCPAD to train Community Health Insurance Agents in Wa Municipal and Sissala West. The contract which outlines the Terms of Reference, was signed on the 23rd of April, 2010.

B. Development of Training Materials

Following the signing of contract, CCPAD worked with NSD, another organization contracted as a Local Capacity Builder (LCB) to deliver similar assignments in other districts schemes, to develop training materials. The first thing was that, a meeting was convened by SNV and attended by the two LCBs to agree on the topics.

The proposed topics were validated in separate meetings held with all the targeted mutual health insurance schemes. CCPAD held separate meetings with the Wa Municipal and the Sissala West schemes while NSD had discussions with Wa West, Nadowli, Jirapa and Lawra schemes. These meetings were very relevant. They allowed the schemes to have fair understanding of the training areas and made meaningful suggestions on which topics required more emphases.

NSD and CCPAD met on three different occasions and developed the training presentations and other materials. The presentations and materials covered eleven (11) topics namely:

- Community Mobilization Strategies

- Participatory Approaches

- Adult Handling

- Facilitation

- Communication

- Advocacy/Networking

- Resource Mobilization

- Health Insurance, it Actors and Processes

- Indigent Identification

- Community Health Insurance Planning

- Record Keeping

As part of the design, we incorporated group discussion, plenary presentations, mock exercise and other participatory tools to make the sessions more interesting and more relevant to the audience.

C. CHIA Training, How It Went

Training of Community Health Insurance Agents was successfully conducted in the Wa Municipal and the Sissala West Districts. In the Wa Municipal, the training took place on the 8th and 9th, and on the 15th and 16th of May 2010 at the scheme's office while in Sissala West it happened on the 24th and 25th of June 2010 at the District Assembly hall. The training was to equip Community Health Agents and staff of the schemes skills in participatory community mobilization and indigent identification. It was also an opportunity for Community Health insurance Agents to Share their experience on community mobilization in their respective communities and allow for real discussion on how to effectively increase enrolment and identify indigents.

Training was delivered in a participatory manner, having participants talk more and facilitators do less. We did this through group discussions, brainstorming, mock facilitation, buzz group sessions, round robbing, open forums, and discussion at plenary.

In all, 170 participants were trained; 56 from Wa Municipal and 114 from Sissala West District. Participants were Community Health Insurance Agents and Scheme staff.

The training was conducted for two days in both districts.

Day 1

Day one was used to know each other better and prepare participants for thinking on how to effectively increase participation in indigent identification and increase enrolment. We therefore introduced participants to participatory approaches, strategies and concepts.

Topics treated on day 1 were:

- Community Mobilization Strategies

- Participatory Approaches

- Adult Handling

- Facilitation

- Communication

- Advocacy/Networking

Day 2

Day 2 of training concentrated on topics that specifically target the role CHIAs will play and how they will do it to bring efficiency into indigent identification and increasing enrolment. It was very easy to have participants linking the participatory concept, strategies and approaches discussed in day 1 to what they are to and how they are to do it. We specifically discussed:

- Resource Mobilization

- Health Insurance, it Actors and Processes

- Indigent Identification

- Community Health Insurance Planning

- Record Keeping

Summary of feedback on each Topic

As expected, participants had different levels of understanding on most of the training topics and therefore presented varied feedback and feedback on the topics discussed. For instance in Wa Municipal, CHIAs did not clearly understand the gate-keeper system in health insurance and did not sensitize clients on it. Clients therefore move right to the Regional Hospital (a referral unit) any time they are taken ill rather than access to health care at the lowest health facility. In the Sissala West, CHIAs clearly misunderstood who indigents were and how they should be identified. What they used to do was to allow communities to present people based on sections to be enrolled as indigents. The community decided how many people should come from each section to make up the number that the CHIA had allocated to them. The table below indicates the methods used and the feedback obtained on each of the training topics.

Table 1: Feedback On Training Topics

S/N	Training Topic	Methods used	Participants Feedback (immediate change)
1	Community Mobilization and Participatory Approaches	• Lecture • Group work • Brainstorm • Buzz grouping • Round Robbing • Plenary Discussion	• Participants have greater appreciation of what community is. They understand that community can be defined geographically or by other defining factors such as religion,

			occupation, sex and age groupings.
			• CHIAs had some level of understanding of community mobilization but did not clearly understand what strategies to employ to enhance participation. Training equipped participants with some participatory tools and methods (community meetings/dur bars, Focus Group Discussions (FGDs), Brainstorm, Round

			Robbing, Buzz Grouping, Question and Answer Sessions, Public Hearings, Laffe Raga, Role Plays and Drama)
			• Participants now appreciate how important it is to effectively mobilize communities for health insurance
2	Adult Handling	• Group work • Brainstorm • Plenary Discussion	• Adult handling was not new to participants but they did not clearly appreciate how important it was in health

			insurance.
			• Participants are more cautious of the challenges in handling adults and understand effective ways of handling their clients to ensure greater participation using the adult handling skills learnt.
3	Facilitation	• Lecture • Group work • Plenary Discussion • Brainstorm	• Participants have been practicing facilitation in their few community sessions that they organized. What they were deficient in

			was the understanding of effective facilitation and how to use it to promote participation
			• The training clearly distinguished between facilitation and teaching, the qualities of a good facilitator, the importance of facilitation and how facilitation can be used to increase participation of community members in health insurance. As a result, CHIAs are

			now more prepared to use facilitation in their activities.
4	Communicat ion	• Lecture • Group work • Plenary Discussion	• CHIAs had an idea as to what communicati on was and the form that exist. • After the discussion participants got to know that communicati on is a two-way system; the message and the feedback. Forms of communicati on, barriers to effective participation, the importance of

			communication and practical ways of promoting effective communication in health insurance at the community level were clearly appreciated by CHIAs.
5	Advocacy and Networking	• Lecture • Group work • Plenary Discussion	• Networking and advocacy were no new terms to participants. They were able to outline some ways they have advocated at the scheme level to have cards delivered within the 3 months

				period. They were also able to indicate how they work with the chiefs and the health workers on health insurance.
				• The training sharpened their understandin g on what advocacy is, advocacy methods and processes, effective way of identifying advocacy issues and how to plan and conduct advocacy.
				• Participants also acquired skills on what networking is,

			importance of networking among CHIAs and other stakeholders and practical ways of strengthenin g networking at the community level.
6	Resource Mobilization	• Group work • Plenary Discussion • Brainstorm • Experience sharing	• Participants understand why resources should be mobilized for health insurance. Some CHIAs were already using innovative ways such as supporting clients to collect stone and sell to contractors while others

			made their community members to engage in dry season gardening just to be able to comfortably pay their premium.
			• The discussions arrived at very important innovations that could be used by CHIAs in their communities to have clients pay premium with less stress. One is the Village Savings and Loans Associations (VSLAs) concept

			which people can raise funds to pay premium. The Village Savings and Loans system is predominant in Sissala West already. Wa Municipal will explore the possibility of instituting it. • The training therefore challenged CHIAs to think outside the box to have community members paying premium without any serious difficulty.

| 7 | Health Insurance, Its Actors and Processes | • Group work

• Plenary Discussion

• Brainstorm

• Lecture | • CHIAs had appreciable level of understanding of the health insurance structure and processes. However, the main difficulty was the gate-keeper system which was not understood by many agents.

• After going through the structure, participants were happy to know that the scheme could support them technically to deliver community sensitization |

			sessions. They were also glad that the scheme was prepared to attend community level meetings to explain some prominent challenges especially those that had to do with delay in the issuance of cards and receipts for premium paid.
8	Indigent Identificatio n	• Experience sharing • Group work • Plenary Discussion • Brainstorm	• Participants showed a good understandin g of the LI on indigent identification and the challenges associated with its

			implementati on in this part of the country. Bottlenecks in identifying indigents using the LI prevent a lot more people who qualify as indigents from being enrolled.
			• The training supported CHIAs to identify practical ways of working with community members and some stakeholders to enroll all people who are qualified as indigents.
			• Some of the ways are; CHIAs will

			exercise discretion in identifying indigents. Also community members would be sensitized to understand the essence of enrolling very poor people as indigents so as to reduce the stigma associated with it.
9	Community Health Insurance Planning	• Group work • Plenary Discussion • Lecture	• Participants did not indicate any fore knowledge of the topic before the discussion. • The participants were very happy to have such a

			tool, as it will enhance participation monitoring and ownership of health insurance activities at the community level.
10	Record Keeping	• Experience sharing • Group work • Plenary Discussion	• Record keeping and data entry is not a problem at the community level. The very complex data is kept at the scheme level • However, there was the need to take participants through some of the formats such

			as the community register and the cash book format to sharpen participants' skills.
			• Treating the topic also emphasized key areas that where CHIAs made mistakes when entering data.

7. Significant Outcomes Of The Training

The training produced very significant outcomes that are relevant for the success and sustainability of health insurance. First of all, Community Health Insurance Agents and scheme staff have renewed spirit to engage communities to increase enrolment especially of indigents. The discussion around the current performance of the scheme have shown that though coverage is high, there is sharp drop in the number of people that are renewing. CHIAs have shown more commitment to working on that.

The introduction of Community Health Action Planning process was another important result of the training. Community Health Insurance Agents initially took activities of health insurance in their communities as their sole responsibility. That posture has affected the way community members perceive the ownership of health insurance. Unlike before, the introduction of Community Health Action Planning has clearly indicated the need for community members to be in the forefront of health insurance. CHIAs only need to provide facilitation for community members to plan, implement, monitor and review action plans to upscale health insurance in their communities.

Training on community mobilization and other participatory approaches has broadened the community engagement toolbox. That has not only provided them innovative ways of engaging their communities for health insurance, but has also given them self-confidence to engage community members effectively on health insurance.

Furthermore, the training on resource mobilization particularly exposed CHIAs to practical ways of mobilizing resources as individual and groups for health insurance. Mobilization of social capital for health insurance is significant in ensuring that every registered member is comfortably renewing membership of health insurance. CHIAs were challenged to think outside the box to find innovative ways of getting community members pay for health insurance without feeling it in their pockets. Specific approach identified was the use of the Village Savings and Loans Scheme (VSLS) approach to get community members mobilizing resources for their own health insurance. In line with that, Community Health Insurance Agents are to mobilize community members into groups and have the scheme supporting them with the necessary logistics to start VSLS particularly in the Wa Municipal. In case of Sissala West, the scheme will hold discussion with Plan Ghana, which is facilitating VSLS to see the possibility of incorporating health insurance into the operations of VSLS.

Another important outcome was the streamlining of the identification of indigents. Indigent identification has been a big problem not just for the two schemes but also in all the schemes in the region. The Upper West Region has been recording the lowest in terms of indigent numbers notwithstanding being the poorest region. The training presented an opportunity for thorough discussion on practical ways of identifying indigents in communities.

8. CHIAs, What They Say About The Training

CHIAs were very impressed with the training in that the context was very relevant and the delivery was a different and better one. Most participants commended the style of facilitation that sought to have participants talking more and being very active in sessions.

They were however some suggestions with respect of the duration for the training. The training was so loaded and stretched participants to the last bit of their energy. Participants believe the training should have been for one week instead of just the two days scheduled considering the volume of content that they had to cover.

That apart, participants also bemoaned their weakness in turning up for the training early. However, some attempted reasons were given.

1. Training was not residential, thus participants had to move from their communities, which of course are quite distant. In some cases, there are no vehicles plying the routes and participants had to relay on motorbikes and bicycles.

2. Also participants got home very exhausted on the first day. It was then very difficult to have participants getting to the training venue on time on the second day.

Direct Statements from participants

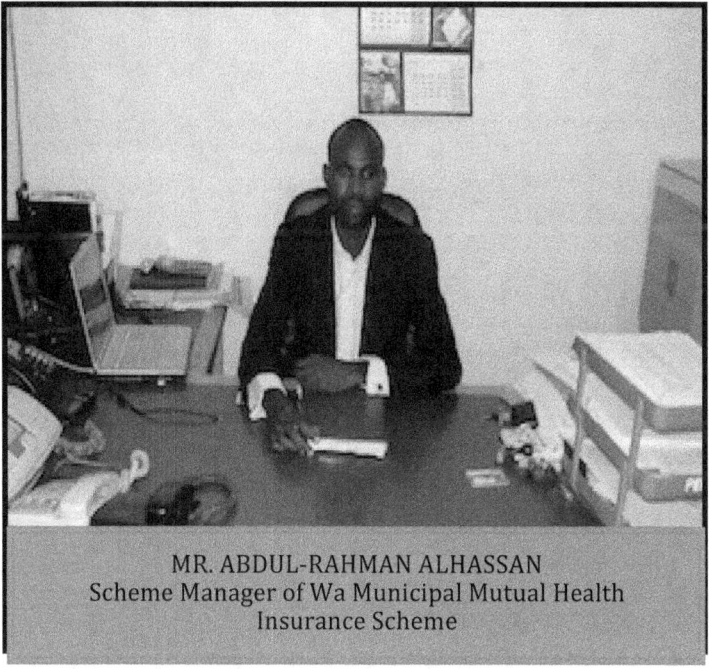

MR. ABDUL-RAHMAN ALHASSAN
Scheme Manager of Wa Municipal Mutual Health
Insurance Scheme

The Scheme Manager for Wa Municipal expressed his opinion about the training.

The training is very useful. It will empower my agents to improve on clients handling. That has been a big issue for us as a scheme. It has also indicated to our CHIAs that engagement of community members should be their initiative. Action Planning is also another great idea. Communities will need to plan health insurance and manage it more or less at their own level. Resource mobilization training was significant. Community members need to be engaged to look elsewhere for resources to pay premium rather than relaying on the pocket all times. We will give CHIAs our support (technical and logistical) to implement some of the innovative ideas that came out of this training. However, we will be contacting CCPAD and SNV for more support in the follow-up activities. In short, the training was impressive.

The Scheme of manager of Sisaala West Mutual Health Insurance Scheme also made similar comments about the training. He was however very excited that the

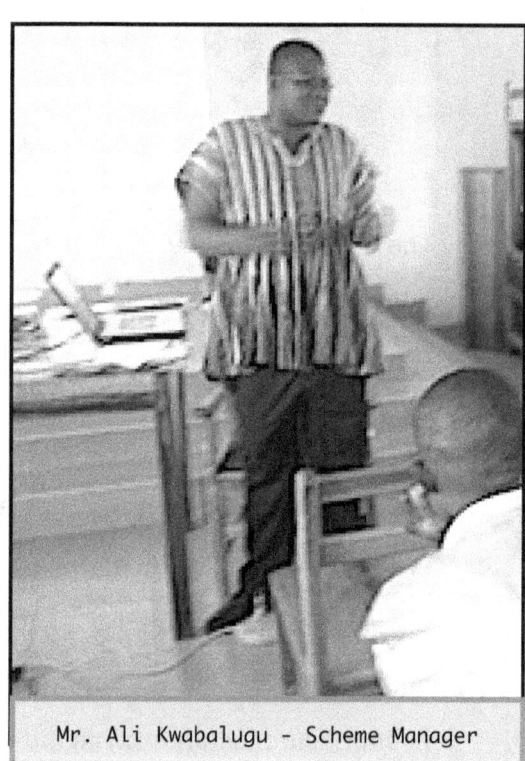

Mr. Ali Kwabalugu - Scheme Manager

issues of who an indigent is and how to identify him/her have clearly been explained. He believes CHIAs will improve on indigent identification.

The Community Health Insurance Agent for Charia was so excited about the training. He indicated that the training was the first ever, in health insurance that allowed participants to freely express themselves and learn. He explained how the training will make their work very easy for them and indicated his readiness to move health insurance beyond the current level. He clearly understood who an indigent was and why that person should be enrolled notwithstanding the socio-cultural barriers such as the stigma around being core poor, which scared many away from accepting registration as indigents. Other participants made similar comments.

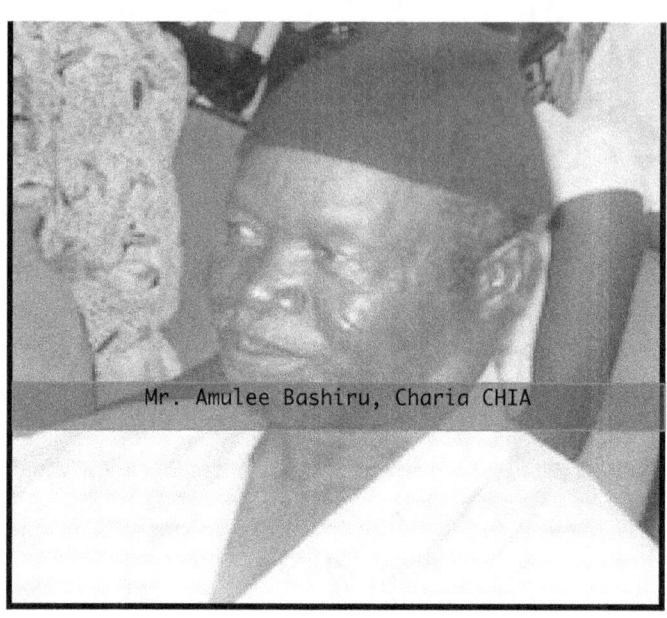

Mr. Amulee Bashiru, Charia CHIA

9. Way Forward

The training is a one-off activity and as such will require a number of follow-up activities by CHIAs, the Schemes and support organizations (SNV and CCPAD).

First of all, CHIAs should be committed to implementing the outcomes of the training and using participatory approaches in their community engagement approaches. How that can be done is to have the scheme playing a monitoring role and providing the necessary backstopping to ensure that CHIAs are able to use the tools.

Secondly, the interest and the excitement about he work of CHIA gathered from the training must not be allowed to wane. It is a very important ingredient in motivating CHIAs to want to do more in health insurance in their communities. Therefore, the scheme should have regular interaction with CHIAs either in the form of community visit or meetings.

Thirdly, SNV as a key partner in health insurance in the region should monitor the implementation of training outcomes. Review sessions could be organized to find out from CHIAs and the scheme where they have reached in the implementation and how that is impacting on their work. Joint field visits could also be made by SNV and the scheme to monitor.

Lastly, the scheme should seek greater collaboration with community level and district level stakeholders such as NGOs, Health, Education and

District/Municipal Assembly to support them in disseminating information on health insurance and engaging community members to actively participate in health insurance activities.

10. Conclusion

Training of Community Health Insurance Agents was a significant move to promote participation of community members in health insurance in order to bring efficiency in indigent identification and improve enrolment. The training focus and the methodology clearly excited participants and satisfied the objective of building capacity of CHIAs on participatory approaches.

It must be stated that, putting the training together was challenging for the schemes in that resources were not readily availably for that. Worse of the two was Sissala West which had very low enrolment. They virtually had to put on hold the training for well over a month to mobilize resources for the training. It would have been very useful to take into consideration the challenges of individual schemes in designing the training.

www.ingramcontent.com/pod-product-compliance
Lightning Source LLC
Chambersburg PA
CBHW070323290526
45791CB00003B/1229